Patient Safety

Stories for a digital world

HAROLD THIMBLEBY with PRUE THIMBLEBY

Dedicated to my father Peter Thimbleby
who would not have died
if the hospital had used a digital infusion pump

"The real data of safety is stories."
— James Reason

"The best way to communicate from one human being
to another is through story."
— Donald Knuth

We tell many stories in this booklet
Stories get our attention and lead to action

Typeset in Computer Modern using LaTeX
ISBN: 978-1-3999-7542-1

CONTENTS

QUESTIONS

INFORMATION

TRUE STORIES

FICTIONALISED TRUE STORIES

THINK LIST

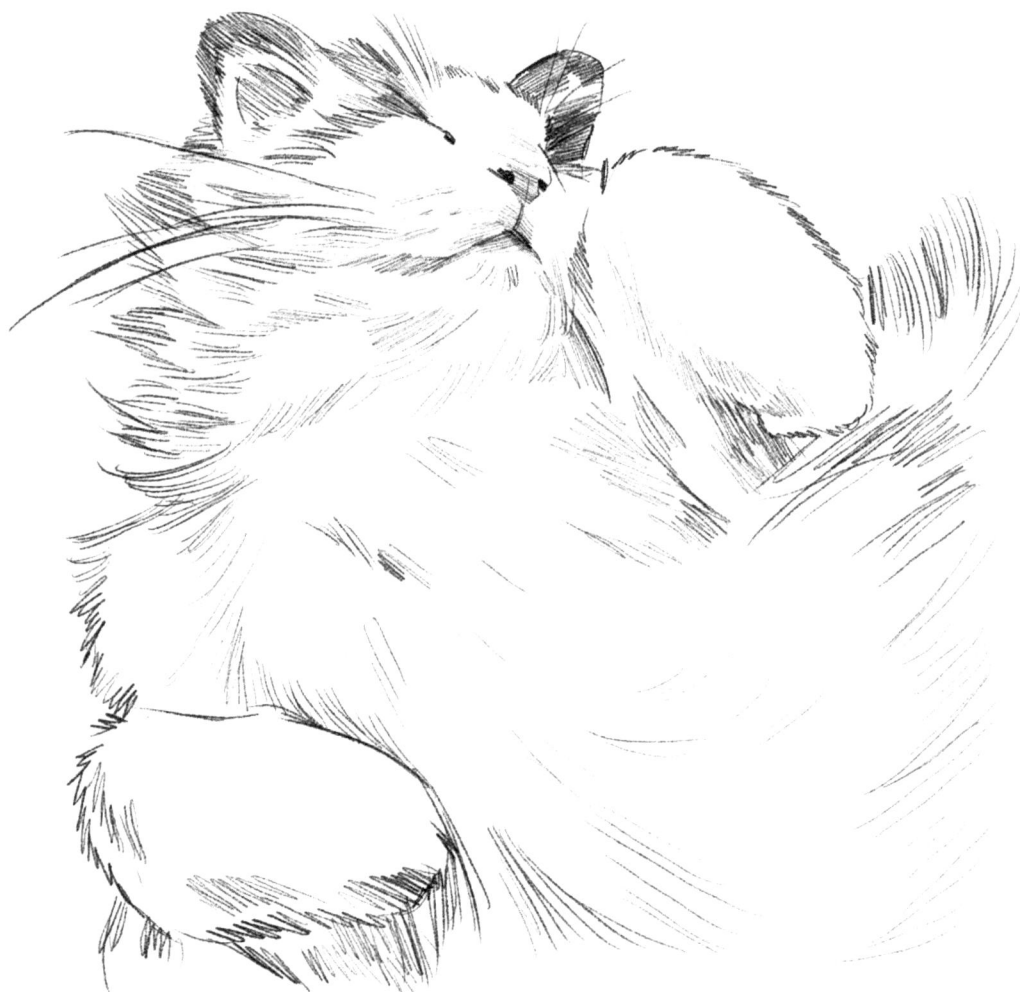

One day, we were eating a meal at the kitchen table. We could hear Po, our new kitten, scrabbling around in his litter tray, scattering litter to try to cover his poo. He proudly walked into the kitchen and jumped up on our table.

Po rolled onto his back, and purred.

As if on command, we tickled his tummy. Aaaaah. He's so sweet . . .

In less than a second, we went from being sensible people, worrying about infection risks and food hygiene, to mindless people seduced by a furry, purring kitten.

***

Driving our uncritical happiness was a cocktail of hormones: endorphins, dopamine, oxytocin, norepinephrine, and prolactin, as we stroked and petted the little kitten.

Our brains, driven by hormones, left us no choice but to feel good. Po purred at the centre of our attention. The world was a happy place!

We both totally forgot all about the bugs at the end of his sharp claws.

Here's the insight: subconscious hormonal excitement makes us overlook problems, like bugs. We call this **Cat Thinking**.

We fall for the same Cat Thinking trap when we enthusiastically buy into the latest digital promises and don't see the problems. It happens in digital healthcare all the time.

Social media apps are designed to make us love them — which makes us want everything digital to be as nice as social media seems to be.

In reality, digital health first has to work with a large complex system involving lots of people. It isn't about how innovative or exciting digital feels, but whether it works, whether it is effective and whether it safely and efficiently supports people — staff, patients, families — in healthcare.

Unfortunately things can and do go wrong in healthcare.

Maybe a patient dies from an overdose, and typically the investigators will say the technology worked correctly, as designed. They therefore think the staff must have caused the problems because digital is wonderful. It purrs, and anyway it was very expensive and it promised to solve all such problems. Sack, discipline, or imprison frontline staff and "the problem's solved" — except it is a misunderstood problem, and it hasn't been solved. Poor system design was probably the key factor.

Most of us are eager consumers of exciting new things, and everything they promise. So we're culturally and hormonally driven to overlook how things go wrong because of poor design and bugs. There are plenty of stories about digital problems and their solutions later in this booklet.

? The British Medical Association says huge numbers of hours are lost to poor digital healthcare. When were you last frustrated with a digital system?

We must start thinking much more carefully and critically. Improving healthcare isn't just a matter of getting exciting new digital systems, like new apps and AI. "New" itself won't fix anything, unless the culture that created and sustained the old problems is improved.

We need to improve the way digital healthcare is designed and regulated. We need improved digital skills everywhere, from developers to procurement to incident investigators. "Unconscious digital incompetence" (which we don't even know we have) must become a thing of the past.

Cat Thinking might sound trivial, but the consequences of such hormonally-driven thinking are very serious. Read this booklet to find out more and what to do about it . . .
Fix IT page 25

Think! Don't get sucked in by exciting technology. Be curious and critical.

IN THE BEGINNING

Back in 2000, I was a professor of computer science at UCL (University College London) teaching and researching how to design computers to be safe and easy to use. Then Nick, one of my students, was run over and ended up in hospital.

I went to visit Nick, and found him on an infusion pump with a Post-It note stuck on it. It said "Don't press this button!" I wondered why not, and as I do research in this sort of thing, I bought an identical pump and studied it.

I was surprised how bad it seemed, but maybe I didn't understand how infusion pumps should be safely and properly used.

So I found an anæsthetist who was interested in safety, and he asked me to shadow him for a week.

In every one of the six operations I attended, something digital failed.

The simplest story is when the ventilator crashed without any warning. It just stopped working. It was literally the blue screen of death from Microsoft Windows.

The anæsthetist had to reboot it and re-enter all the patient details all over again, so the patient wouldn't suffocate.

Worryingly, the anæsthetist thought this was normal and didn't realise things could be better. He did not report the incident, so neither the regulators nor manufacturers ever found out.

Fix IT pages 35 & 38

Since that experience with infusion pumps and ventilators I have continued to research digital health, to see how it can be made easier to use and safer. My research culminated in my book, *Fix IT: See and Solve the Problems of Digital Healthcare*.

Fix IT is published by Oxford University Press. Rather late in the day they got in contact with me about a missing picture. They were worried that there was a page with a caption but no picture to go with it. There was just a large blank gap. What did I want to do?

I explained. On one page there is a box listing all the things an anæsthetist needs to know to qualify. Once an anæsthetist passes they can, for instance, use a ventilator.

On the opposite, facing, page there's a box containing everything a programmer is required to know before they can develop ventilators.

It's completely empty — which was intentional — as there is no requirement that medical device programmers are qualified in any way or must have studied anything relevant. Neither the patient nor the anæsthetist has any reason to trust the ventilator. All the anæsthetist's skill in pressing the right button at the right time can be undone by the ventilator's poor programming making it do something unexpected.

Fix IT page 39

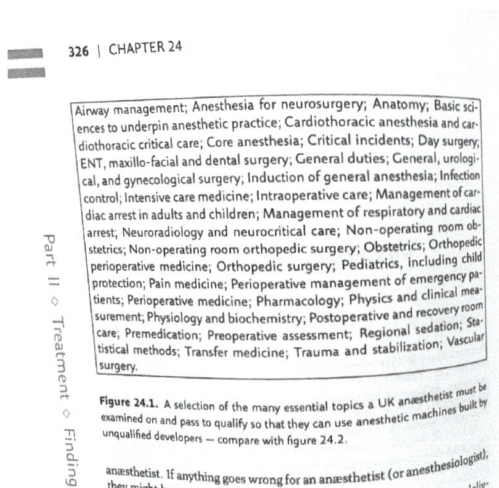

Airway management; Anesthesia for neurosurgery; Anatomy; Basic sciences to underpin anesthetic practice; Cardiothoracic anesthesia and cardiothoracic critical care; Core anesthesia; Critical incidents; Day surgery; ENT, maxillo-facial and dental surgery; General duties; General, urological, and gynecological surgery; Induction of general anesthesia; Infection control; Intensive care medicine; Intraoperative care; Management of cardiac arrest in adults and children; Management of respiratory and cardiac arrest; Neuroradiology and neurocritical care; Non-operating room obstetrics; Non-operating room orthopedic surgery; Obstetrics; Orthopedic perioperative medicine; Orthopedic surgery; Pediatrics, including child protection; Pain medicine; Perioperative management of emergency patients; Perioperative medicine; Pharmacology; Physics and clinical measurement; Physiology and biochemistry; Postoperative and recovery room care; Premedication; Preoperative assessment; Regional sedation; Statistical methods; Transfer medicine; Trauma and stabilization; Vascular surgery.

Figure 24.1. A selection of the many essential topics a UK anæsthetist must be examined on and pass to qualify so that they can use anesthetic machines built by unqualified developers — compare with figure 24.2.

anæsthetist. If anything goes wrong for an anæsthetist (or anesthesiologist), they might h...

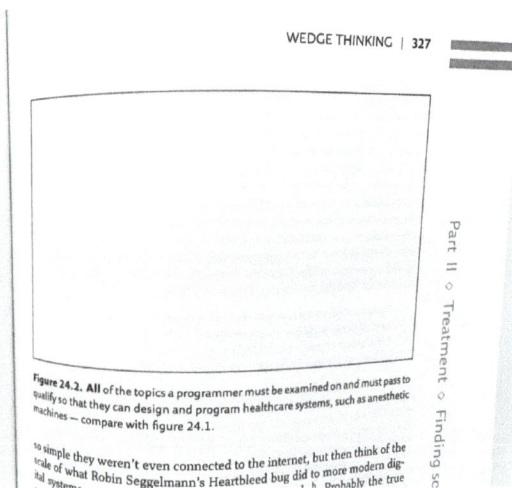

Figure 24.2. All of the topics a programmer must be examined on and must pass to qualify so that they can design and program healthcare systems, such as anesthetic machines — compare with figure 24.1.

so simple they weren't even connected to the internet, but then think of the scale of what Robin Seggelmann's Heartbleed bug did to more modern digital system...

4

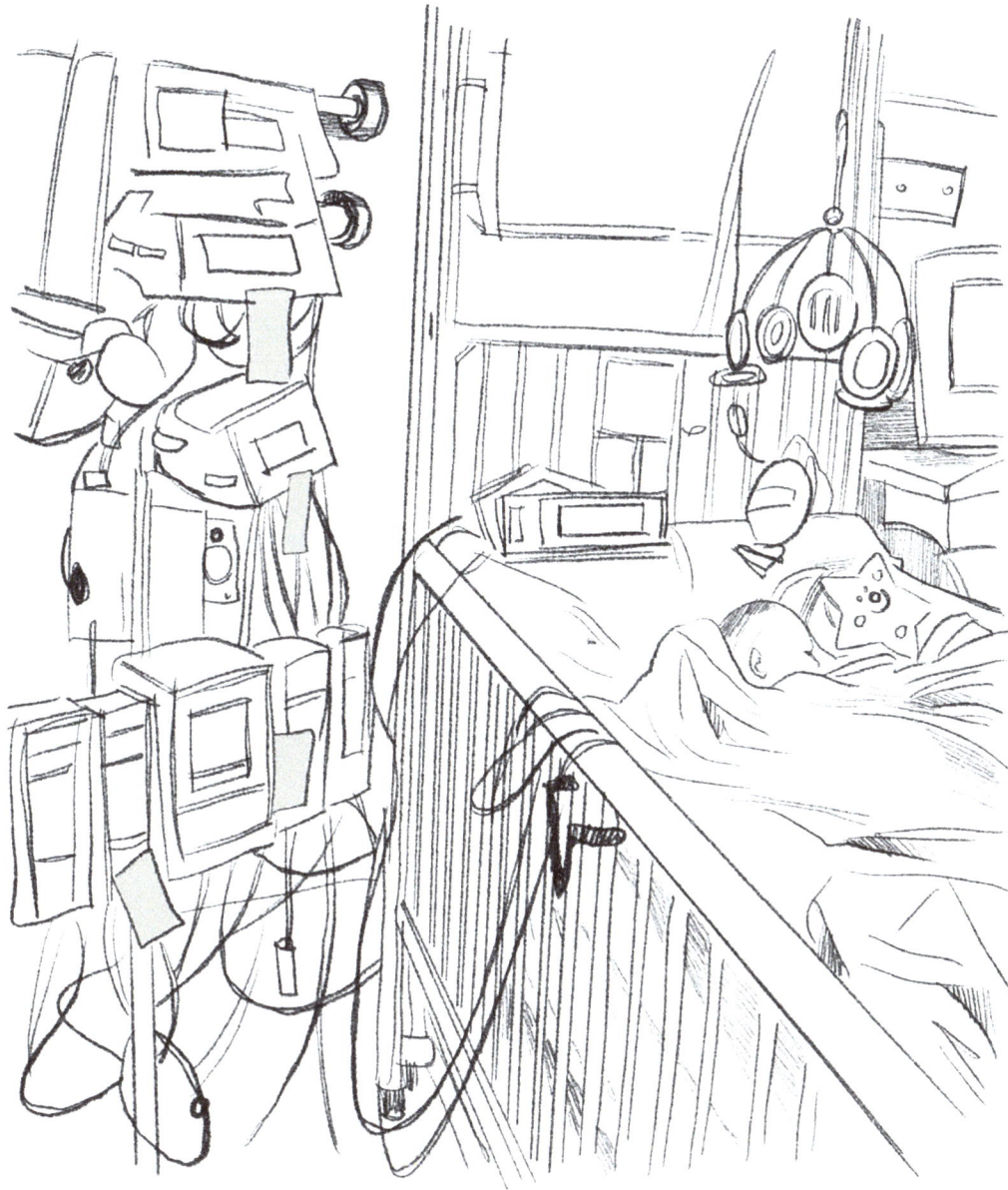

Post-it notes used on infusion pumps   *Fix IT* page 39

If you want to be an electrician and wire up a hospital, the law says you must be qualified and up to date with the regulations. Yet if you want to build medical devices, ventilators, diabetic glucose meters, medical apps, X ray machines, GP appointment systems — anything digital in healthcare — then you don't need any qualifications at all.

That's why the ventilator in the story crashed. It was designed and developed by people who were out of their depth. It's impossible to assess people's programming skills without qualifications.

Nobody is required to have digital qualifications for IT procurement or IT management either, so the ventilator was bought and used by people who had no idea it was poorly programmed. It should have been a lot better.

Think! Qualifications for software developers in healthcare should be required by law, just like qualifications are for clinicians.

"My heart leapt with joy! We had been trying for a baby for several months and now my period was three weeks late and the test was positive. The wave of joy was followed by a twinge of anxiety which came from having watched my brother grow up with all the challenges of having Down Syndrome. We had decided to have the Down Syndrome test and then we could plan what to do.

Fortunately, the test was all clear, and I began to relax and look forward to meeting our baby.

With less than a month to go everything was going to plan.

The baby's room was all ready. The excitement was building.

Then, and I will never forget that moment, I read in the local paper that the software for testing for Down Syndrome in our area had errors in it, and many women's results were inaccurate.

The floodgates of emotion opened, and when my partner came home from work, I was a blubbering wreck on the floor. Suddenly I had no idea what the rest of my life would be like . . .

Fix IT page 33

Right from the first days of 2000, midwives worried about getting unusual Down screening results. Something was wrong. In April a midwife coordinator rang the Immunology Department, and spoke to Mr M. She wasn't just querying one odd result, but months of odd patterns of results.

Mr M believed it could wait for Mr K, who was on leave. Despite the standard incident reporting procedures, Mr M did not record the midwife's phone call.

Over a month later, after getting more phone calls, letters, and other messages expressing concern, Mr K finally realised there was indeed a problem.

Of the 7,000 mothers potentially affected by incorrect calculations, Mr K told the Inquiry that he had identified 150 calculations that had moved from low chance to high chance. Two terminations are known to have been carried out because of incorrect screening reports, and four babies with Down Syndrome were born to mothers who thought their tests put them in the low-chance group. A hotline was set up, run by midwives, to support concerned mothers.

Fix IT page 500

? Apart from the problem gradually escalating while nobody took it seriously, what was the underlying cause of the problem?

The Millennium Bug is what had gone wrong, and the programmers and other technicians hadn't realised just how serious that was. They thought all the individual problems were unrelated, and that they were not significant. Besides, they had had a Millennium Bug workplan, and they didn't expect any computer problems.

Yet their Millennium Bug code was messing up thousands of patient ages, which were an essential part of the Down Syndrome screening calculations.

An unqualified programmer at the Northern General Hospital in Sheffield had taken short cuts that turned out not to work, resulting in a computer system having bugs that caused clinical chaos.

The problem was initially not taken seriously by technicians and clinical staff. Eventually, a major incident was reported, and an inquiry was set up to find out what had gone wrong, and to report on changes that must be made.

The inquiry report included advice from a consultant chemical pathologist, who wrote an analysis of the original computer code and provided new code, which itself was buggy (defective). Furthermore, the pathologist knew and admitted that his new code did not handle leap years correctly, despite the year 2000 (the year of the incident) itself being a leap year. The inquiry's new, recommended code was thus as bad as the original, indeed arguably worse because it came with the official inquiry's authority as a corrected solution.

Here, then, was a hospital developing, implementing, and investigating its own computer systems from scratch without any professional software engineering oversight — and making many mistakes.

BUGS AND MORE BUGS

The Millennium Bug. A computer needs to know the age of the patient when Down screening is done, as it uses their age to help calculate the significance of the laboratory test result.

I was born in 1955. Throughout the 20th century, a computer could work out my age very easily. For instance, in 1980, code could do the simple sum 80 minus 55 to work out my age as 25 years old (give or take a few months).

In the new millennium, all such computer programs' simple age calculations went wrong. My age in 2000 would have been worked out as 00 minus 55, which would have meant I was apparently **minus** 55.

Not only did the Down program have the Millennium Bug messing up patient ages, but it didn't do a "sanity check" that the patient ages it was using made some sense (like being numbers between 10 and 100), so it went ahead and calculated bad test results from crazy ages calculated by bad code.

Any critical system should be programmed to report and block wild results being used. This one didn't.

In addition, the patient's age was not reported on any screening results sent to the midwives, so the midwives were not able to see when incorrect ages had been used.

In short, there was no professional error checking anywhere.

Historically, millions of developers made elementary mistakes creating Millennium Bugs worldwide. It's important to remember that, although the Millennium Bug itself is old history, it's remains an alarming warning of the scale of poor design practice, which continues to affect today's digital healthcare. The following short list is the tip of the iceberg:

- In 2011 the NHS's National Programme for IT (NPfIT) became the world's largest single IT failure. NPfIT was cancelled after wasting around £20 billion, and very little was learned.
- In 2018 a bug in a GP system resulted in 150,000 patients being affected by a data breach.
- In 2020 nearly 16,000 COVID-19 cases were lost due to naïve Excel programming, and around 50,000 people were lost to contact tracers.
- In 2020/1 Cambridge University Hospitals released 22,000 patients' information by mistakenly including them in an Excel spreadsheet. This major error was only noticed three years later!
- In 2023 a hospital trust failed to send out 24,000 letters to patients and their GPs after they became lost in a new computer system.
- In 2023 a hospital trust had 927 Datix reports raising concerns about the ironically named "Surrey Safe Care" system: one patient died and over 30 others suffered harms.
- In 2023 updating patient information in Magentius Software's Euroking system overwrites other patient data. Attempts to correct patient records can result in further corruption. All problems affect patient safety, and can raise false evidence of staff misconduct or tampering with patient records. The manufacturer promotes Euroking as a "market-leading maternity solution" to "improve safety and clinical care during the maternity process."
- In 2024 despite over 24 years of publicity, a Y2K bug repeatedly made American Airlines treat a 101 year old former nurse as a 1 year old baby and didn't provide the wheelchair she booked. Even with unprecedented worldwide awareness, elementary but critical bugs still persist!

Almost every healthcare system still has problems of being slow, needing another password, not being interoperable, needing upgrades, ignoring critical errors, and worse. England's official independent patient safety investigation body, the Health Services Safety Investigation Board (HSSIB), has recently said that **digital failures are among the most serious issues facing hospitals**. **Computer failures are found in nearly every investigation HSSIB carry out.**

Dr Rosie Benneyworth, interim HSSIB head says, "**We have seen evidence of patient deaths as a result of IT systems not working.**"

Poor digital healthcare is a widespread, international problem. Every week there is another case of digital failures in the news, yet politicians and leaders everywhere continue to set ambitious goals with seductive promises for digital health without prioritising the quality of the digital engineering competence.

Fix IT page 19

Think! You need digitally-qualified specialists as part of incident investigation teams.

A HOSPITAL-WIDE PROBLEM

" I was standing in my kitchen and checking my work emails before I cooked the family dinner. That is when the bombshell hit. The email said I was not to go into work the next day. I was suspended.

I sat down at the kitchen table trying to take in what was happening. Trying to make my eyes focus and read the detail of what the email was saying.

I loved my job as a nurse on the cardiac ward. I loved the banter with the patients. How could something have gone so wrong as to lead to suspension? The email outlined that I was being accused of falsifying glucometer readings. We always had a number of diabetic patients on the ward, and we recorded their blood sugars regularly. I couldn't believe that I had somehow recorded them wrongly.

I rang my friend who I worked with. I was embarrassed, but I needed to talk to someone. She had just had the same email!

It turned out that over 70 nurses had been suspended. That helped — to not feel I was on my own. To not feel like the one black sheep that had let my patients down.

I thought long and hard about how I took and recorded the readings. I really couldn't remember ever making up numbers or forgetting to record them. My brain went over and over it, and when they said things would be easier if I pleaded guilty and admitted my errors I really didn't know what to do. If I pleaded innocent, but was found guilty, I would get a harsher sentence, maybe even go to prison. They said there was lots of computer evidence that showed I was guilty.

How could I argue against that?

In 2016 I was asked to be an expert witness in a court case involving two nurses who were being prosecuted for criminal negligence in their care of diabetic patients. The case was part of a large incident in the Princess of Wales Hospital where 73 nurses had been suspended because computer records showed that they'd failed to do their job professionally. The police prosecuted some of the allegedly worst offenders.

Before a criminal trial, the defence and prosecution meet to review the case and see if it really needs to go to court. I was baffled how 73 nurses could all be so bad in exactly the same way, so I asked how the prosecution could believe all 73 nurses had made the same mistakes, when there are far simpler explanations like computer error, cyberattacks, or even an IT person with a grudge? The prosecution replied that all the nurses were in it together.

The case went to court, with two nurses in the dock. I was cross-examined almost every day, and ridiculed by the prosecution. Who was I to claim that a system made by a major international company, Abbott, was unreliable?

One day I said something that was too technical for the prosecution, who decided to call Abbott's Chief Engineer to respond to my technical points. When the Chief Engineer testified, he happened to say he'd visited the hospital. I prodded the barrister in front of me, and told her to ask "what did he do?" The Chief Engineer said a bit more about what he'd done. I asked the barrister, "when did he do that?"

I told the barrister: that's exactly when a lot of data vanished. Soon the judge intervened, himself examining the Chief Engineer. He then said the court would be adjourned while he wrote a ruling.

The judge read his ruling to the court. He said the prosecution had wasted everyone's time, and benefitted nobody. He ruled that the computer evidence was of no value, and asked the prosecution what they wanted to do . . .

The prosecution admitted they no longer had a case. The judge called the jury in, and told them there was no case to answer. The jury foreman rose to tell the court that there was no case to answer.

The judge said, "Release the prisoners."

A HOSPITAL-WIDE PROBLEM

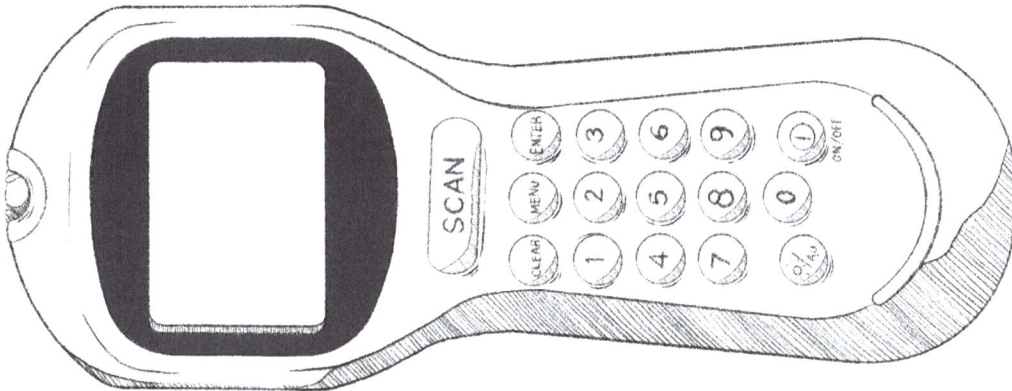

Abbott glucometer as used in the Princess of Wales Hospital

Fix IT page 92

? What were the problems? The Princess of Wales Hospital had problems with their computer records. They called in an engineer to sort out the problems. It became clear in court that the engineer had **really** sorted the problems out, by deleting the problematic data. Later, the hospital relied on these "sorted out" computer systems to provide evidence that nurses had failed in their standard of care. It didn't cross anyone's mind that the computer evidence was unreliable, even as they suspended one nurse after another.

The scale of the problem became so large the police got involved, and it became a criminal investigation.

The mindset that the nurses were to blame became entrenched, and because there was a criminal investigation nobody would talk openly about anything.

It's worrying the hospital did not detect that any data had been corrupted. It didn't notice an insider job deleting data, so how would it have noticed if a cyberattack corrupted data? It looks like it was not managing its systems professionally.

It's even more worrying when you realise that the same and similar systems will be in use in thousands of hospitals around the world with similar lack of monitoring.

Once a case like this reaches the criminal court, a "legal presumption" in the UK makes it very hard for people to defend themselves. In law, the presumption is that computer evidence is correct.

It thus becomes almost impossible for defendants to challenge computer evidence because, since the evidence is presumed to be correct, how can you find out any reasons why error logs, documentation or even program code should be disclosed for your team to review?

We are focussing here on recognising the problems of digital health, but of course there are many amazing things that digital brings to health too. In the book *Fix IT* there is a whole chapter focusing on success stories, one of which is included in this booklet on page 23.

Fix IT page 416

Think! Be slow to blame staff. Ask: could computers, devices, or records be unreliable?

A COUNTRY-WIDE SCANDAL

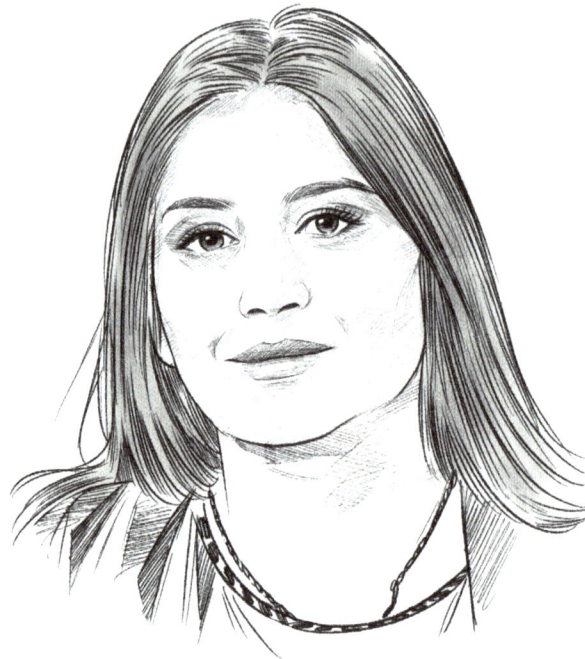

Seema Misra became a post office operator in West Byfleet, Surrey, in 2005. Over the next two years she had attempted to balance her books, borrowing money and transferring takings using the Horizon accounting system provided by the Post Office.

Seema regularly reported her problems to the Post Office Helpline — several times a week, and each time she was told to "roll over" the accounts or balance them with her own cash.

Finally, she failed to keep her head above water.

After an audit of her accounts found a discrepancy of £74,000, she refused to plead guilty and was prosecuted by the Post Office. During the trial, she found she was pregnant.

It came as a complete shock when she was convicted of theft and false accounting. Seema collapsed in the dock when the judge read her sentence, sending her to jail. She was ordered to pay compensation to the Post Office.

The media called Seema a "pregnant thief." Her husband, Davinder, was beaten up by locals, who accused them of coming to the UK "to steal old people's money."

Jarnail Singh, the Post Office's senior criminal lawyer, celebrated Seema's conviction. He sent an email to Post Office executives saying "It is hoped the case will set a marker to dissuade other defendants from jumping on the Horizon bashing bandwagon." He added: "Through the hard work of everyone . . . we were able to destroy, to the criminal standard of proof, every suggestion made by the defence."

In prison, Seema was put on suicide watch.

Seema says, "If I hadn't been pregnant I would have definitely killed myself."

In fact, Seema's £74,600 shortfall was caused by bugs in the Horizon computer system.

It was not until 2021 that Seema's conviction, along with 38 other postmasters' convictions, was overturned by the Court of Appeal. The Court of Appeal ruled that her prosecution by the Post Office was abusive, an affront to justice, and an affront to the conscience of the Court, a rare and extraordinarily severe ruling. It had taken eleven years to prove Seema's innocence.

Seema is one of more than 900 post office operators wrongly prosecuted for fraud, theft, and false accounting.

Fix IT page 508

A COUNTRY-WIDE SCANDAL

The Post Office Horizon scandal is basically the same story as the nurses suspended over alleged negligence. The Horizon scandal is in this booklet because it shows how serious digital problems are widespread, widely ignored, and ongoing.

An organisation gets an expensive digital system, which promises to revolutionise how work will be done. In fact, both Fujitsu (for the Post Office's Horizon system) and Abbott (for hospital blood glucometers) claimed their systems would reduce error.

Then someone is found apparently to have made some mistake. Stolen money or not performed a test on a patient. Such things happen, regrettably. There are procedures to follow.

A few days or weeks later, another guilty person is identified and blamed. And, again, procedures are followed. And so on.

Soon the organisation realises its reputation is at stake. The media gets interested. The organisation knuckles down as the number of "guilty" people rises.

Nobody wants to stop and think — or admit — that their computer systems may be unreliable. In the courts, the computer evidence is presented as infallible.

The defendants are told the evidence against them is overwhelming. "Do you remember **exactly** what you did several years ago? Well, the computer does."

So they are sure to be convicted, and should plead guilty to reduce their sentence.

Then, in court, the law backs up the Post Office. It is presumed that the computer evidence is correct. This presumption means that the prosecuting organisation does not need to justify to the court why it thinks its computer evidence is correct.

In the Horizon case, it's clear that at some point the Post Office knew the evidence it was using was wrong, and it then went into a major cover up.

The official home page for the Post Office Horizon IT Inquiry where lots more details can be found is
https://www.postofficehorizoninquiry.org.uk

The Post Office relied on a detail of British Common Law: computer evidence is presumed correct.

This legal presumption was recommended by the Law Commission. There's good evidence that they, the people at the top, also misunderstand computers.

There are huge differences in the Post Office and Princess of Wales cases.

The Post Office Horizon IT Inquiry is finding many examples of the Post Office's willful misrepresentation of facts about Horizon. The Court of Appeal ruled that the Post Office's convictions were achieved by a serious abuse of the Court system. The Post Office prevented a fair trial, and the Court of Appeal called the Post Office abusive.

In contrast, senior staff at the Princess of Wales Hospital believed the computer evidence and never realised otherwise. It seems surprising, though, that they hadn't the curiosity to investigate why so many nurses apparently failed in exactly the same way.

The Post Office Horizon IT Inquiry has been shown some of the computer code inside Fujitsu's Horizon system. Here's a very short example.

The idea of this bit of Horizon code is to make the value of d negative. You would imagine it would say something like "set d to $-d$."

Instead, it says "if $d < 0$ then set d to the absolute value of d, otherwise set d to d minus twice d." If you wanted to make something very straight forward obscure and error-prone, hard to understand, and hard to debug — this is a good way to do so. It's coding to be ashamed of, and has no place in professional code. It's just irresponsible.

Professional programmers will also notice this peculiar code misses an important opportunity to check there are no errors (e.g., it's possible $d = -d$ even when $d \neq 0$).

Lots of Horizon code has other bizarre problems, but the bugs are too intricate to explain here as the code is so confused.

HEADS IN THE SAND

" As I pushed open the door of the hospital, I could immediately see that something was wrong. There were people milling around the foyer looking like they didn't know where to go. The volunteers on the reception desk were on the phone. One was writing out a big notice. I saw the word "cyberattack."

It was 14 May 2021, and I was working as a doctor in Dublin, Ireland. We were already in the middle of a pandemic, and a cyberattack would make things go from bad to worse.

And it did go from bad to worse. The chaos that followed was indescribable.

There were no lists of patients for my clinic. I couldn't access any medical records online. I couldn't print labels for blood tests.

One of my patients needed a scan to see if his cancer had shrunk. I had to go down to the scan department to view the scan because they couldn't send it up to me. But then I couldn't tell the patient whether he was getting better because I couldn't access his last scan to compare it.

All computer screens were down — nothing was working.

We had to shut the radiotherapy unit whist we worked out how to safely calculate and administer treatment. Patients kept arriving as we had no way of cancelling appointments because we couldn't even access the booking lists and find out who had appointments.

That night we had an emergency meeting to pool ideas on how to keep operating safely. We started using WhatsApp to communicate and send images. The criminals demanded $20 million. They said they already had 700Gb of our patient data that they would be releasing.

The stress of caring for people and keeping them safe is indescribable.

Fix IT page 214

The HSE, the Health Services Executive, is basically the NHS of Ireland. It has over 130,000 staff who are dependent on connected and reliable digital systems.

The Conti cyberattack started on 16 March 2021. On 18 March, somebody opened a phishing email, which included a malicious Microsoft Excel spreadsheet. The user's access rights let the Conti cyberattack in. The cyberattack at first spread silently.

There were in fact several earlier occasions when people noticed the beginning of the attack, but these were not declared a cyber incident, so opportunities to start fixing the problem before it had seriously escalated were missed.

The full cyber onslaught detonated on 14 May. Because Conti encrypted data, staff across Ireland lost use of every IT system, including patient information systems, clinical care systems, laboratory systems, financial systems, payroll, and procurement systems. Even monitoring sterilisation. Everything went down.

Email and even phone lines went down too. There was no way to communicate with HSE's national centre. Everyone had to revert to pen and paper to work and continue patient care, or improvise using their own phones with apps like WhatsApp.

The chaos lasted over six months.

Given Conti happened during the pandemic, there was a terrible load on staff. The cyberattack management team formally brought in Occupational Health because staff mental health had become a critical issue in managing the recovery. Clinical Indemnity had to be provided to doctors, nurses and midwives, because there were no patient records and nothing worked.

It took till the end of September 2021 to sort it out, when all servers were considered decrypted, and with most, but not all, applications restored back to use.

Cyber-training for staff is essential. However, front line staff should not have to learn how to compensate for poor and unsafe design — more can be done by manufacturers in the first place, and in healthcare behind the scenes by IT support.

Ironically, in Ireland, the people who did best during the cyber-attack were those who still relied on paper instead of digital. Although going paperless is often held up as the ideal, paper will remain an essential fall-back for the foreseeable future.

HEADS IN THE SAND

The gang who developed the Conti cyberattack used off-the-shelf tools, readily available to any hacker, to create it. It was basic stuff. It could have been much, much worse had the hackers had any serious plan. Their attack didn't spread from HSE's internal systems to external cloud systems, for instance.

The hackers had encrypted data, so making it useless. Maybe because they realised their attack had had a terrible effect on an entire nation and they were out of their depth, they soon released a decryption key. It wasn't perfect but made recovering data a little easier. Malicious hackers could have deleted data (and data on backups), or, worse, corrupted it so that patient records were wrong. Malicious hackers could have targeted particular patients: famous patients, or types of patients the hackers didn't like. Hackers could have changed blood results or drug regimens — or anything.

Fortunately, the Conti attack was technically trivial stuff.

? HSE, like everyone else, had already had experience of cyberattacks like WannaCry. The question arises why had HSE not kept up maintaining and developing defences against cyberattack?

The Conti attack exposed that the Irish national health service was operating on fragile IT with a system that had evolved without much thought, rather than been designed for resilience and security.

It wasn't just the computer systems, but the management systems too: management had no professional cybersecurity expertise. The report into the Conti attack says "The HSE also had only circa 15 full-time equivalent ('FTE') staff in cybersecurity roles, and they did not possess the expertise and experience to perform the tasks expected of them."

It was a tall order for inexperienced people to recover from a cyberattack, especially when the attack had broken the obvious means to communicate with all staff.

It's an international problem, and needs international collaboration.

You can explain a cyberattack away by saying it was caused by criminals, or possibly by under-trained staff who had not done enough cyber-awareness training. All true, but a more strategic understanding is that the digital systems were inadequate. They had backdoors that shouldn't have been there. The manufacturers should have continually maintained the systems, with updates routinely applied by local IT staff.

There should be no legacy (out-dated) systems in healthcare.

Manufacturers should have warned and helped transition to more modern, safer and more secure systems — after all, they built in the original weaknesses that the criminals exploited.

Manufacturers' warranties and contracts typically exclude digitally-related liabilities. On the contrary, we should contractually require manufacturers to guarantee that their systems are, as far as reasonably practical, free of safety-related errors throughout their lifecycle.

If a manufacturer won't stake their business on the quality of their products, don't stake patients' lives on their products!

Fix IT pages 298 & 313

In the UK, the Health and Social Care Act requires compliance with standards, like DCB 0129 and DCB 0160. These standards require a clinically-qualified safety officer, risk assessment registers, and more, but don't require digitally-competent work nor technically diverse independent oversight.

As the DCB standards unfortunately don't go into technicalities of digital safety, so when a healthcare organisation doesn't fully understand digital — which, sadly, is too often, as this booklet makes clear — it may assume its nominal compliance with any such standards is sufficient. It will be unaware that it is not managing digital risk safely or effectively. (The Further Reading, on page 27, gives a case study discussing the complexities behind the "simple" case of NHS Numbers.)

It would therefore be helpful to supplement using the DCB standards with more prescriptive industrial standards that include technical guidance, such as the authoritative *NASA Software Safety Guidebook* available at https://standards.nasa.gov/standard/NASA/NASA-STD-871913

Think! Continually check cybersecurity compliance, including software updates, following national best practice and alerts.

RaDonda Vaught was familiar with the BD Pyxis, an automatic drug dispensing cabinet, at Vanderbilt University Medical Center (Tennessee, USA). In December 2017, RaDonda needed some Versed, a sedative, to help an anxious patient, 75 year old Charlene Murphy, relax and have her MRI scan without worrying.

To get Versed out of the drug cabinet, you would type VE, and select Versed from the screen showing everything starting with VE. Once a drug is selected, a drawer with several boxes will open, and the right box will pop open automatically, and you take the drug out.

But this particular day things didn't work like that. RaDonda couldn't find any Versed. As was routine in the hospital, RaDonda did an "override" to get a larger list of drugs, to show more options starting with VE. It was common practice to override the cabinets, as they were so hard to use. Some reports say there was a "persistent software problem."

Interestingly, the hospital had reprogrammed its drug cabinets to accept short 2 letter abbreviations to make them easier to use, despite 5 letters being widely recommended for safety reasons.

RaDonda entered VE again, a drawer opened, and a box popped open.

RaDonda took the drug out and gave it to Charlene. Unfortunately, the drug wasn't Versed, and Charlene died soon afterwards because she'd tragically been given Vecuronium, which is a paralytic.

The Versed was actually stored in the cabinet only under its generic name, Midazolam, so typing VE would never have found it.

Note that the first 5 letters of Versed and Vecuronium are different. Following best practice would have blocked RaDonda's error and nothing would have gone wrong.

RaDonda reported the error. She was fired from the hospital, arrested and prosecuted. She was found guilty of gross neglect of an impaired adult and negligent homicide.

Fix IT page 172

The case triggered a widespread outcry. The American Bar Association says, "A robust culture of safety relies on self-reporting and transparency to drive process improvement, and criminalising errors instead foments blame and creates fear."

Paul Curzon tried out a magic card trick on me. "Pick a card . . . any card," he'd say, and then he'd identify the card I had secretly picked. He kept on doing it! Everyone watching was laughing, but I just couldn't see what he was doing to keep catching me out.

Paul was deliberately, and very successfully, fooling me by carefully controlling my attention, memory, and expectations.

Magic like this proves how easy it is to manipulate things so that people will predictably make the same mistakes.

Magicians do it for entertainment. Conmen do it to cheat you. Email phishing can trick people out of money — or a whole country out of having working healthcare.

Digital healthcare tricks us by accident, but unfortunately accidental misdirection is as good as tricking us deliberately. A situation needing a workaround or override, for instance as RaDonda needed, sets up the user to be misdirected and fall for a trick.

The psychology of attention and predictable error, which are used to trick us in magic, can be turned right around into the positive science of Human Factors: how to manage and avoid error, how to avoid being tricked — mistakenly or otherwise — into unwanted surprises. Crucially, Human Factors (and reliable Software Engineering) can help designers avoid building misleading digital systems.

Yet medical systems used in hospitals accidentally perform "tricks" on staff every day. Staff miss critical details because they are misdirected by a toxic mix of clinical pressure and poor design.

Fortunately, healthcare staff are professional, and usually they very soon notice problems. But sometimes, they have no idea they are being tricked, and the consequences may be catastrophic for patients.

Just like I was surprised and confused by Paul's card tricks, staff trying to use complex devices — like automated drug cabinets — can be surprised and confused about what happens. This makes them very easy to blame when mistakes happen.

Incident investigators, too, are often unaware how often poor digital design, whether poor Human Factors or poor Software Engineering, is the real "root cause" of error.

AS IF BY MAGIC

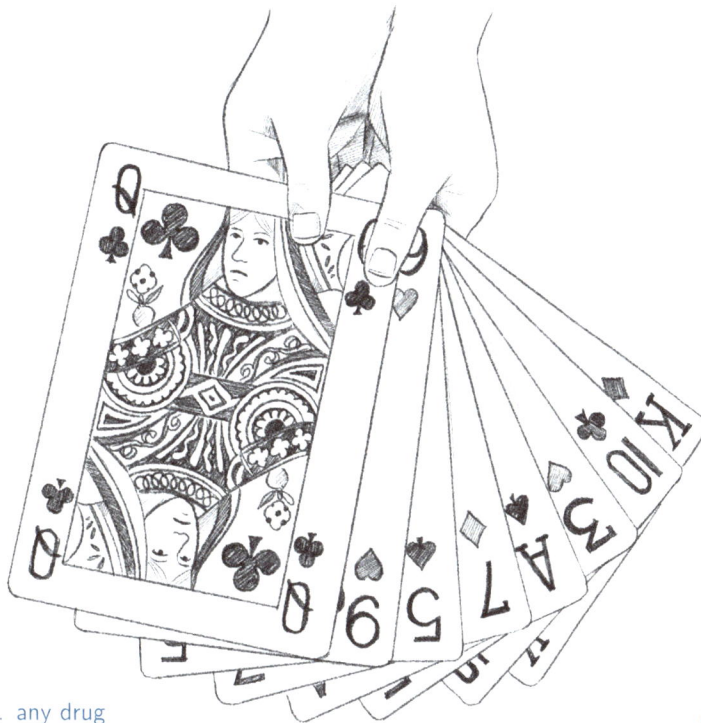

Pick a drug ... any drug   *Fix IT* page 262

" I am the head of pharmacy at a large American hospital. Digital medicine and prescribing is a really exciting area for innovation and improving efficiency. Our hospital is at the cutting edge.

I've been in lots of meetings discussing AI and robots. We had a campaign to get approval to buy the latest technology. Last month, we were one of the first hospitals to install a $7 million pharmacy robot.

The new robot promises to eliminate human error. But only today, a doctor entered a dose of 160 milligrams per kilogram of patient weight, when it should have been 160 milligrams full stop. So the intended dose of 160 milligrams was multiplied up by the patient's weight. This was a very large overdose.

The wrong dose wasn't noticed by the system, but was packaged up by the robot, and the patient was given this dose by a nurse who was just doing what the robot told her to do.

Very sadly, six hours later, the patient fitted and stopped breathing.

This has brought us down with a huge bump — it's tragic that $7 million of the latest AI and robots isn't sufficient to eliminate error.

Fix IT page 126

? Why wasn't such a dangerously wrong dose noticed by the hospital's new robot? In fact, clinicians had been overwhelmed with irritating computer error messages interrupting them all the time, so the hospital medical center had decided to disable many alerts. Having disabled alerts, of roughly 350,000 medication orders a month, there were now "only" 17,000 alerts a month. Unfortunately, the mistake described above was not spotted because it was one of the blocked alerts.

Think! Understanding Human Factors is essential for developers and for incident investigators.

In 2021 a strong candidate applying for a training post in anæsthetics in the UK was rejected by the digital recruitment system, Oriel. The candidate was surprised to find out they were "unappointable." After an investigation into their complaint, it was found that 34 more candidates had been affected as well.

Separate Excel spreadsheets to record candidates were created by people across the country. The spreadsheets varied depending on who had created them, which made them hard — and error-prone — to combine into a final master spreadsheet. The inquiry into the incident also found that few people developing the spreadsheets understood the behaviour of Excel's VLOOKUP function, which had been used in the spreadsheets.

Fortunately, nobody was harmed by this interoperability fiasco, but the story is a warning for anyone developing digital systems, including spreadsheets, that will be used for clinical purposes.

? What was the problem?
The main reason why digital things go wrong is that people — whether clinicians, administrators, investigators, technicians or developers — don't notice when technicalities start going over their heads.

People drift into creating applications (here, Excel spreadsheets) that require professional software engineering skills to do well. Because they aren't software engineers, they don't notice the transition from what seem simple, obvious ideas to needing professional skills as things scale up. They likely don't understand the very basic software ideas, like specifications, assertions, invariants, testing, pair programming, code review, user interface design (UCD), user experience (UX), and iterative design, or why these principles are essential to develop systems reliably.

The same trap swallows up developers too. It's very easy to program and "make things appear to work," but it's **very** hard to make things work safely under the complex conditions of healthcare.

We also need to be careful to spot the cowboy developers (like in Babylon Health) who routinely go beyond their limits while claiming to have the experience and skills.

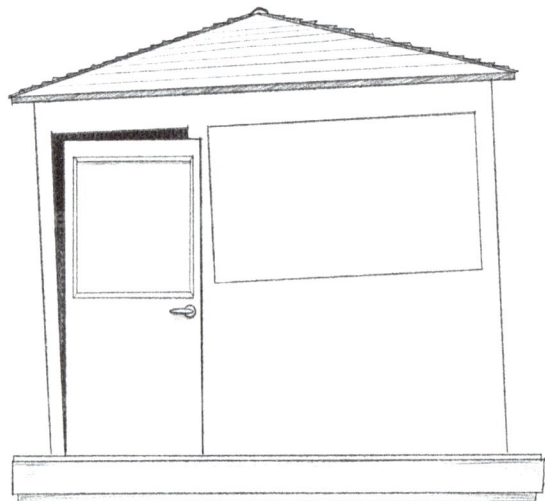

I am good at DIY. In 2017 I built a garden office, but I made a rookie mistake that cost a lot.

I paid some builders to lay the concrete foundations. I watched them pour the concrete — I even helped them make sure it was the right size and perfectly level.

When the concrete had set, I built the office, complete with its red tiled roof to keep the rain out. I then started to fit the details, and found out that the door wouldn't fit. In fact, everything was slightly twisted. The office was like the Leaning Tower of Pisa.

I had just assumed the foundations were level. But unfortunately, when the builders tamped down the concrete, the frame sank down in one corner.

I hadn't double-checked.

I had to dismantle the whole thing, and get the builders back to re-lay the concrete more carefully. Then I had to start all over again.

Like DIY itself, DIY programming is very popular. It's very easy to start a DIY digital health project, but if we make a mistake we don't notice and so don't fix it, our code may harm thousands and put staff in prison.

Fortunately, there are ways to avoid and correct mistakes. A first step is to recognise our limits — for instance, no self-aware DIYer would contemplate building a tower block!

The best way to recognise our limits is to get educated, and the best way to prove that's happened is through qualifications.

RECOGNISING AND AVOIDING PROBLEMS

A common way to cause an error is, ironically, to correct an error you **do** notice.

Imagine you are to enter 5.5 mg as a drug dose on an infusion pump. Unfortunately, you accidentally press the decimal point twice in a row as maybe the key bounces. You probably realise you typed 5.. , so you press the delete or backspace key, to correct the number back to 5. , so you can continue with pressing the 5 key. In the end you'll have entered 5.5 .

Unfortunately, the patient gets 55 mg not 5.5 mg, because almost all devices delete **both** the decimal points. Worse, if this bug results in an incident, the device's log will show what **it** did, not what **you** told it to do.

Fix IT page 177

According to the *Daily Mail*, Arsula Samson died because a "blundering nurse" entered a ten times overdose.

No error was found with the infusion pump (its logs wouldn't have shown anything insightful). Investigators ruled the death was due to "individual, human error." The coroner's verdict was accidental death to which neglect contributed.

The hospital's action plan saw medical staff retrained, and new infusion pumps and software brought into all wards "to reduce the risk of error." If expensive training, new pumps, and software were needed then the original system must have played a critical part in inducing the tragic error.

Fix IT page 71

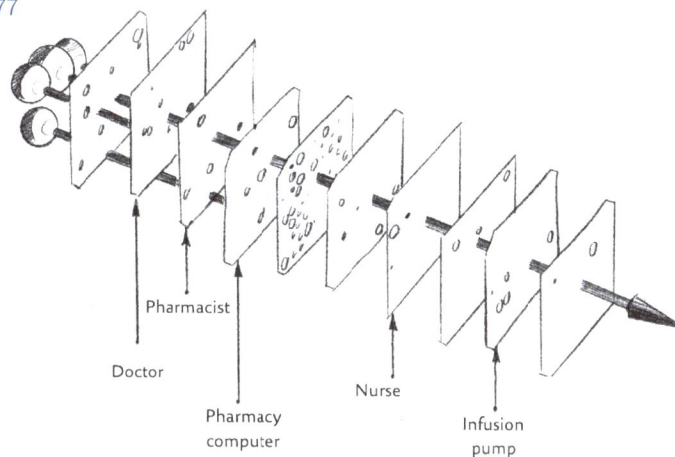

Swiss Cheese showing different members of a team

Fix IT page 60

As this booklet makes very clear, we must never assume digital works reliably. It follows that **all** health work needs multidisciplinary teams that include clinical expertise **as well as** qualified digital expertise — which includes Human Factors, user centred design, and more.

It's not just a matter of implementing things right as a purely technical exercise, but the right thing must be implemented! For that, engaging users (both patients and staff) and collecting real-life evidence is absolutely critical using UCD, UX, iterative design, and so on, otherwise new systems will just cause new problems.

Post-implementation, teams need to continue to work together to improve the digital and spot problems. And the teams need to keep evolving, because digital itself is changing very rapidly.

Fix IT page 105

Swiss Cheese, with its image of slices of cheese with holes that let errors through, is often used to help understand how harms are never caused by just one failure: **everything** has to fail, not just a scapegoated member of staff who takes the blame.

More constructively, each slice of cheese represents a different defence against errors turning into catastrophes. Digital, done properly, is important as it's a very different sort of cheese that can catch and stop errors that humans easily miss.

Digital experts in healthcare teams will also be able to spot system weaknesses that clinicians are likely to miss. Equally, clinicians in digital teams will stop clinical errors being built into new digital system designs.

Think! Know your limits, and work in a qualified interdisciplinary team.

Deaths and illness around childbirth had always been a fact of life until 1847, when Dr Ignaz Semmelweis noticed that his hospital wards had a higher rate than the nearby convent hospital. He set out to find out why. What was he doing wrong?

Semmelweis started collecting statistics. He noticed that his wards had fewer sick patients in the summer. But why? He realised that in winter his doctors attended autopsies to learn about anatomy, then went straight back to the wards. In summer they didn't do this so often.

Semmelweis speculated something was getting back to the wards from diseased bodies in the morgue. He instituted hand washing. His intervention soon reduced maternal death from around 20% to 2%.

Unfortunately, Semmelweis met a lot of resistance to his ideas. Doctors didn't like being told they might be the cause of illness. After all, Semmelweis had no real theory why his ideas worked.

A real explanation had to wait until Louis Pasteur developed germ theory, which at first only explained fermentation. The Scottish surgeon Joseph Lister then connected germ theory to putrefaction and disease. Lister realised that antiseptics would destroy germs causing disease, and his success as a surgeon soon became famous. Healthcare was persuaded.

Antiseptics prevent but don't cure disease. Effective cures had to wait for antibiotics, which Alexander Fleming discovered when he identified penicillin in 1928.

Antibiotics are now widely used to treat infections. But in turn, using antibiotics is creating new problems in this invisible world of bugs. Bacteria evolve, and become resistant to antibiotics. Some antibiotics are thus losing their power, which can be catastrophic for infected patients — it's a new global health threat. Guidelines are being developed so antibiotics are only used when they are effective and don't increase antibiotic resistance.

Bugs that cause disease are invisible, and for thousands of years, people could only speculate about illness. Most people just accepted disease.

Eventually, Ignaz Semmelweis worked out a cause of disease, but he met considerable resistance from his colleagues.

Digital healthcare is a new intervention, affecting all areas of healthcare. Digital health has hidden bugs.

Managing digital bugs doesn't require antiseptic procedures; it requires computational thinking. Unfortunately, just like theories of infection in the nineteenth century, computational thinking meets resistance.

Like Semmelweis's colleagues, we resist being told we may be wrong. Moreover, as cat thinking shows, the excitement about digital itself makes it much harder to think about its limitations and weaknesses. Why would we have bought that expensive AI system if it wasn't going to be an effective system?

Just like early ignorance of bacteria, antiseptics, and antibiotics meant that curing disease was almost impossible, ignorance of computational thinking makes it almost impossible to recognise, talk about, or to address the problems of digital bugs.

? What does **computational thinking** mean?

We haven't defined computational thinking in this booklet. We haven't defined antibiotic either.

You take for granted that to understand antibiotics you need some medical training. It's the same with computational thinking: to understand computational thinking you need computer science and software engineering training.

Chapter 13 in *Fix IT* is all about computational thinking.

There are parallels between **antibiotic resistance** and **digital failure**.

Just like the discovery of antibiotics was revolutionary, and antibiotics were first seen as a "magic cure," so, too, people promote digital as a cure-all solution to many of today's healthcare problems. But it's counter-productive to try to solve problems by getting more or newer digital systems — digital transformation — without stopping to ask: Will it be better? Will it be safe and effective? When is enough enough? We won't know unless we understand the underlying computer science.

Think! Computational thinking is the right approach to understand digital.

LEARNING FROM THE PAST

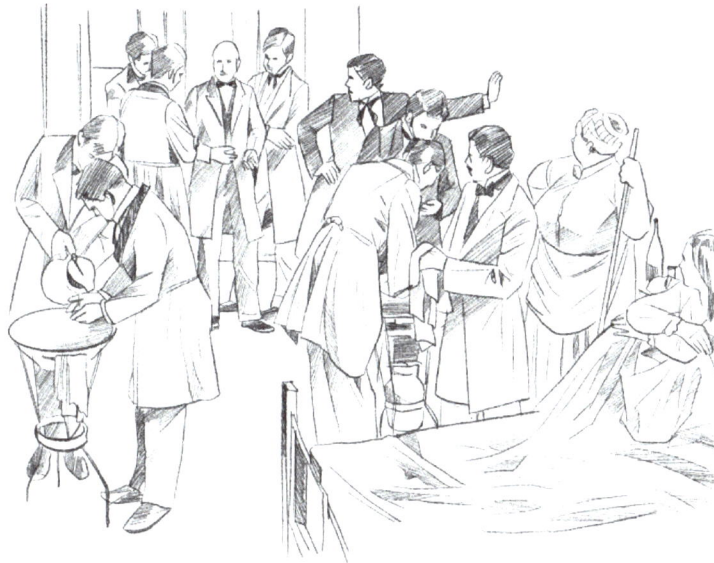

Dr Semmelweis's students washing their hands in his ward   *Fix IT* page 15

Medical device and system manufacturers often complain about regulatory burden — the cost to them of complying with even the current regulations around digital healthcare.

I remember a manufacturer saying that if they followed regulations to the letter, their innovative systems would be so delayed they'd be obsolete by the time they reached the market. I wondered, if things are going to get obsolete so quickly, why would anybody want to spend any money on them?

We wouldn't generally go along with such arguments for drugs — we'd first want to know drugs are safe and mostly free of side effects before they are marketed.

Pharmaceutical companies rarely complain about regulatory burden. They employ highly qualified chemists, often post doctoral, and microbiologists to develop and test new drugs. They take regulation in their stride.

Inexperienced developers use what's called a "happy path" to test their systems. They simply check that things work as they are supposed to work. They can now tell everyone that it works exactly as it's supposed to work — implying any problems are your fault. But the happy path means they didn't check for possible failures.

Competent developers instead test all possible paths where their systems are and aren't used as they are supposed to be. This is very hard, as there are an overwhelming exponential number of ways of using things in unexpected ways. Developers who want to do thorough testing therefore use sophisticated computer tools.

AI, of course, makes safe development **very** much harder — so at least carefully check contracts to ensure manufacturers don't deflect responsibility for safety.

In response to the serious problems of quack doctors, the UK Medical Act 1858 required doctors to be formally registered to practice.

In the same year, some peppermints were accidentally made with arsenic taken from an unmarked barrel instead of from an adjacent barrel of sweetener that wasn't labelled either. The error poisoned more than 200 people, killing 21, mostly children. The deaths led to criminal trials, but the court record says, "The only really criminal thing in the whole affair was that the law could not touch the practice of adulteration . . ." The tragedy thus triggered the Pharmacy Act 1868, which required drugs to be labelled, written records to be kept, and that only qualified pharmacists could sell drugs. There was opposition from many pharmacists over the details; tighter regulation had to wait for the Dangerous Drugs Act 1920.

What will it take before we start regulating digital health, and AI in particular?

Think! We should accept regulating digital — systems, developers, and support — just like we accept healthcare regulation.

SAFETY FIRST

My Dad died from an over-infusion.

A nurse had left a drip running unattended, and Dad went into cardiac failure from too much fluid. It would very likely have been better if Dad had been on a digital infusion pump that had been programmed to stop at a preset maximum dose.

Here's a picture of me having an infusion of rituximab, using just such a digital pump. It was a long process. My dose needed adjusting throughout the day.

I was glad that the type of infusion pump they used with me, an Alaris GP, has up $\triangle$ and down $\triangledown$ keys to adjust the infusion rate. Our research shows that $\triangle/\triangledown$ keys are about twice as safe compared to numeric keys for entering drug doses.

Our research has also shown that you can halve the "out by ten" error rates of numeric keys by better design ("out by ten" errors often happen with the decimal point getting in the wrong place).

Put another way, if you are using a poorly designed system, the design itself will cause its users to make errors.

Fix IT page 412

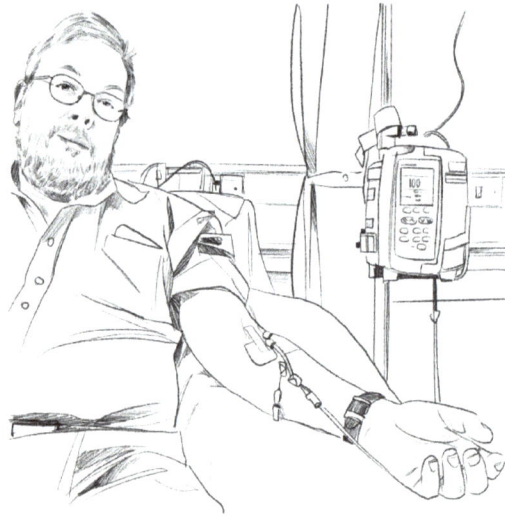

? Digital devices vary enormously in quality, ease of use, safety, and in environmental impact. How does anyone know what a good robot, AI, or infusion pump is?

How can hospitals choose and buy the best and safest equipment? How can people make good decisions? It's tempting to try to buy the cheapest, but running costs are a big factor. Every time an infusion pump is used, new lines are required — and these are often proprietary, only fitting the particular make of infusion pump. This causes "lock in" thus limiting choice. When a contract is set up to buy thousands of pumps over the next ten years, various deals will be done to balance and manage the short and long-term costs.

The procurement process rarely considers the long-term safety or usability, because nobody knows what anything's safety or usability is. They just assume these devices are safe and usable. Indeed, manufacturer's descriptions like "easy to use" or "eliminates error" mean nothing without rigorous evidence.

When we buy tyres for our cars, we have a very similar problem. We want the best tyres, but we don't want to pay over the odds. Some tyres are safer than others, but we have no idea which. Some are clearly cheap re-treads, whereas some are made by reputable manufacturers, sometimes with household names.

The European Union noticed this problem, and decided that we, the customers, needed some help. Tyres now have rating labels, covering stopping distance, noise, and fuel economy. When you buy a tyre you can now see how good it will be.

Fix IT page 401

Think! We need more digital health research and better adoption of research — we need to be evidence-driven.

SAFETY FIRST

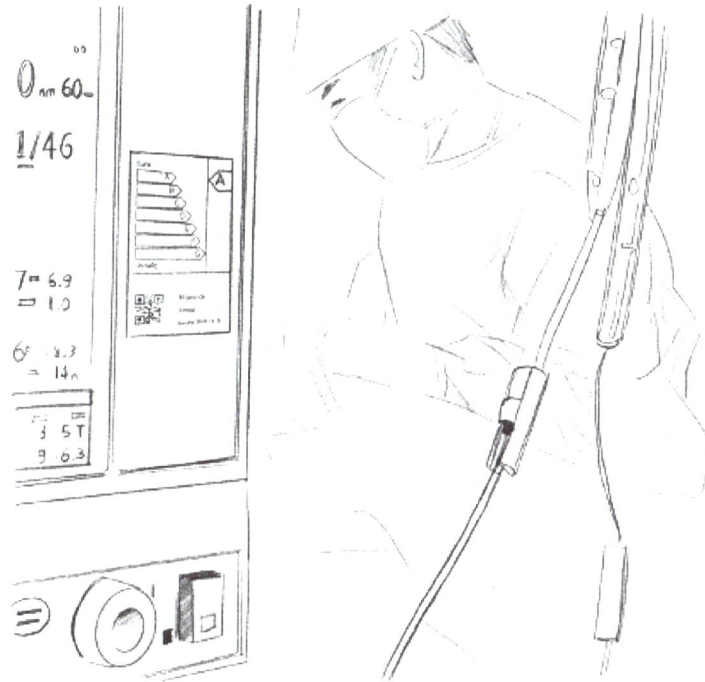

If we took digital safety seriously, safety labels would prominently show how safe and usable every device and system was.

Ratings would combine several measures, such as the results of a bag of standard experiments with real and simulated users, just like car safety tests. The device illustrated in the (imaginary) picture above is 'A' rated.

The safety label in the picture also has a QR code on it, which would quickly provide relevant information about the device. The QR code would lead to a web page that provides access to the device's configuration, serial number and software version, and, ideally, its logs as well.

Staff and patients would all be more aware of how safety depends on quality equipment. Organisations would buy safer equipment. Staff would choose to use safer equipment. Patients would benefit.

Fix IT page 405

There are similar styles of labels for rating the energy consumption of fridges, cookers, and washing machines. Not only do these labels help us know how to buy better products, but they have also improved the quality of products that manufacturers make.

Because efficiency labels help customers see quality, manufacturers who make more energy efficient fridges sell more fridges. So manufacturers now compete to make even more efficient fridges.

In fact, now, as fridges have energy ratings that are far better than the original A rating, the ratings have had to be adjusted to account for the higher standards. Everybody benefits.

It'd be nice if that sort of improvement happened in digital healthcare too.

We already require electrical safety labels (from Portable Appliance Testing, PAT testing) on everything plugged in at work, even though hardly anyone is harmed by electricity at work. So surely digital safety labels are more important?

Fix IT page 402

Think! We need safety ratings to inform procurement. Manufacturers will then make safer and safer systems.

GETTING BETTER

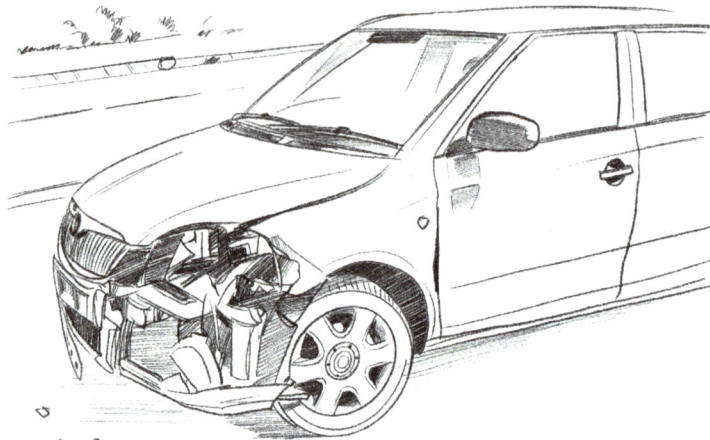

The day before he got married, our son Isaac asked to borrow our car, a silver Škoda Fabia. Well, of course he could!

About an hour later, the police telephoned to say there'd been an accident.

Isaac had collided with another car. The other car had flipped over, ending up in a ditch on the other side of the road.

Shown above you can see how our car looked after the accident. It has a crumple zone at the front, which has crumpled. The air bag also went off, and it saved Isaac from injury. This is what crumple zones and air bags do: they absorb energy in crashes, and save people.

There are many safety features in modern cars that are harder to see, like the seat belts, the ABS brakes, the "crash box" — the rigid frame to protect the passengers — and more. Manufacturers like Škoda are keen to promote their cars on the quality of their safety features.

Car manufacturers today want drivers to survive car accidents, or, better, to **avoid** accidents. If your tyres and brakes are good (and properly maintained) you can stop quickly in a controlled way. You will never have an accident at all if your car stops in time before it hits anything or anyone.

Despite the speed of Isaac's crash, and the damage to the two cars, Isaac and the people in the other car all walked away uninjured.

Safety technology works.

The deeper point is that errors will happen, but they need not lead to harm.

Fix IT page 17

? If Isaac had been driving a 1960s car, at the speed the cars hit each other, he'd likely have died, like in the awful picture below. What changed to make cars safer? What can digital healthcare can learn from industries, like cars and aviation?

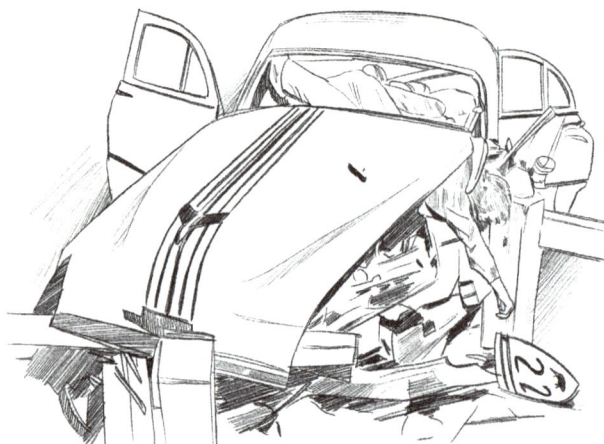

GETTING BETTER

NCAP, the New Car Assessment Program, started testing car safety in 1979, and has been instrumental in making cars safer.

Car manufacturers now appreciate NCAP because it helps them promote how safe their cars are.

People who buy or sell cars want NCAP ratings because they help them negotiate and think clearly about safety and quality.

NCAP is so successful, it's gone global (see www.globalncap.org). What can we learn from NCAP's success to help improve digital healthcare quality?

NCAP has a mission statement, and by changing NCAP's "safer car" focus into a "safer digital healthcare" focus we would get a powerful mission statement for digital healthcare.

Car engineering is a professional field, but, as this booklet has shown repeatedly, digital healthcare isn't. As digital healthcare is way behind car safety, here are three extra points that NCAP didn't need to mention . . .

1. Provide digital healthcare **qualification frameworks** so digital competence can be measured and forced to improve.

2. Once there are qualifications, it must be a **legal requirement** that developers are appropriately qualified and accredited.

3. Digital qualifications and professional accreditation must be developed and regulated through a new competent **professional body** with external oversight.

Fix IT page 467

> **Think! We need a new organisation with statutory powers to set digitally-competent standards and lead a Digital Health Safety Program.**

Jason Maude's story — Good digital saves lives!

"My story starts when Isabel, my three year old daughter, became ill with chickenpox. We took her to the GP, but she got worse, and that evening we took her to the emergency department (ED), and again it was shrugged off as normal chickenpox.

She continued to get worse at home. We went back to the ED, and she was seen by a paediatrician, who looked at her and said, "Oh, she looks a little bit dehydrated." And the nurse who tried to take her blood pressure said, "Oh dear, the blood pressure machine looks as if it's not working properly."

About ten minutes later Isabel's eyes started rolling, and she went into multi-system failure, and crashed. Then it was just chaos.

From that point on, the NHS worked beautifully. The crash team was good. And she was transferred that day by the intensive care retrieval team to St Mary's Hospital, London.

But it needn't have happened.

We decided to create a digital tool to help clinicians put together a differential diagnosis to help clinical reasoning. If you think there are at least 10,000 diseases in the world, it's just impossible for anybody to remember how all those diseases present. And that's what computers are really good at — computers are good at going through mountains of information very, very quickly, and coming up with a shortlist.

So the tool, which we called Isabel, first became available in 2001 — and it worked. When the clinicians tried it, they put in classic cases, and a good list of possible diseases came up.

One of our clients published a paper called "Isabel to the Rescue!" . . . They were close to losing a patient. They decided to use Isabel, and it prompted them to think of brucellosis, which they hadn't thought about. They asked the patient. And, yes, she'd been eating homemade cheese in Mexico. They actually said, "You know, if we hadn't used Isabel, we wouldn't have thought about that — we'd have lost the patient."

Isabel is now used worldwide. Isabel is available for clinicians, and also as a free-to-use web-based symptom checker for patients. It helps patients understand the possible causes of their symptoms, and also directs them to more information and care. See www.isabelhealthcare.com

Fix IT page 431

THINK LIST

? What can we do?
Recognise the problems that need solving
Look through the key points below
Choose your priority for action
Share this booklet . . .

1. Don't get sucked in by exciting technology. Be curious and critical. (p. 3)

2. Qualifications for software developers in healthcare should be required by law, just like qualifications are for clinicians. (p. 5)

3. You need digitally-qualified specialists as part of incident investigation teams. (p. 7)

4. Be slow to blame staff. Ask: could computers, devices, or records be unreliable? (p. 9)

5. The legal presumption that computers are reliable urgently needs correcting. (p. 11)

6. Continually check cybersecurity compliance, including software updates, following national best practice and alerts. (p. 13)

7. Understanding Human Factors is essential for developers and for incident investigators. (p. 15)

8. Know your limits, and work in a qualified interdisciplinary team. (p. 17)

9. Computational thinking is the right approach to understand digital. (p. 18)

10. We should accept regulating digital — systems, developers, and support — just like we accept healthcare regulation. (p. 19)

11. We need more digital health research and better adoption of research — we need to be evidence-driven. (p. 20)

12. We need safety ratings to inform procurement. Manufacturers will then make safer and safer systems. (p. 21)

13. We need a new organisation with statutory powers to set digitally-competent standards and lead a Digital Health Safety Program. (p. 23)

14. We need to prioritise building a new generation of highly skilled digital engineers who can work in or with healthcare to build safe digital healthcare systems. (p. 28)

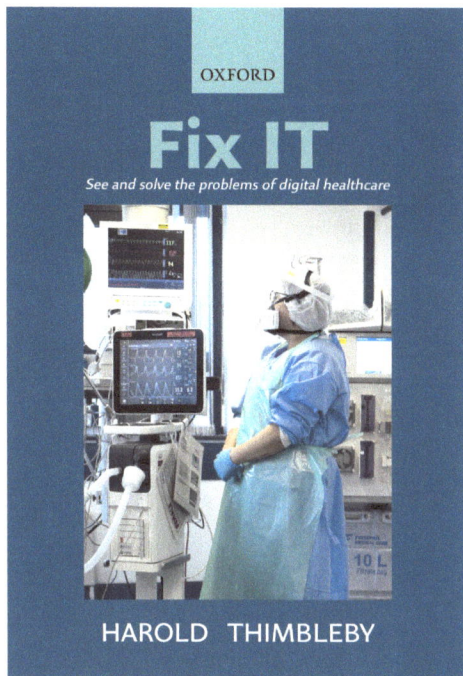

This booklet is based on Harold Thimbleby's book *Fix IT*, which won the British Medical Association's General Medicine book award.

The judging panel said:

> *Fix IT* is such an important book. Our ability to help patients is so reliant on IT and digital solutions. It has the broadest appeal and has achieved something quite impressive. It is not just medically-focused in presenting solutions. A real strength is that it takes examples from outside of healthcare and translates them into healthcare. It should be read by all healthcare staff.

Harold Thimbleby, *Fix IT: See and Solve the Problems of Digital Healthcare*, Oxford University Press, 2021.

The Fix IT prize

In collaboration with the Royal College of Physicians, we have launched an annual prize for digital innovation, **The Fix IT in Healthcare Prize**. The prize rewards excellent innovations in digital healthcare, which help solve the problems described in this booklet, particularly digital initiatives that have improved, or promise to improve, patient safety and staff well-being within the NHS or healthcare internationally.

More details are available from the Royal College of Physicians web site, www.rcplondon.ac.uk, under Funding & Awards.

CHECKLIST FOR WHEN THINGS GO WRONG

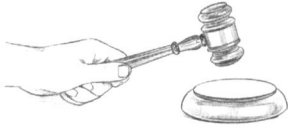

If you end up in a disciplinary hearing, or in litigation, here's what you should consider . . .

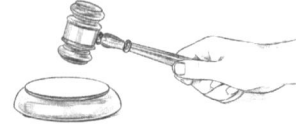

1. You are not alone. Talk to people. Try to find out if other people have had similar experiences — if so, suspect the system, not the people.

2. Check out the NHS Just Culture — for example, it says "Are there indications that other individuals from the same peer group, with comparable experience and qualifications, would behave in the same way in similar circumstances?" — if so, this would be a likely sign of digital problems! (See further reading.)

3. It is important to talk to a competent expert. Although Expert Witnesses are available for court work, a good place to start is to get in contact with your local university Computer Science Department, and talk to someone — maybe a PhD candidate or Research Assistant — who is working in usability, safety, cybersecurity, or dependability.

4. The freely accessible database *MAUDE – Manufacturer and User Facility Device Experience* has details of millions of medical device issues, and may be relevant to your situation. Search online for "FDA Maude."

5. Require the disciplinary panel or your prosecutors to provide the documents listed below. Where these items won't or can't be provided, everyone should treat evidence with appropriate caution. Your friendly expert (see point 3 above) may need to modify or extend this list, depending on your circumstances.

   Note that in a court case, a judge can order disclosure of facts to an Expert Witness if the organisation is not prepared to provide the documents or access to the systems to determine the facts yourselves.

   (a) A copy of the actual computer-readable evidence (not a paper printout) that they are relying on — so you or experts can analyse it. It must be examined by experts before anyone agrees that the system has produced correct output, and what its significance is.

   (b) Copies of independent certification to the relevant international standards that the digital systems are reliable, and adequate for evidential purposes.

   (c) Evidence of the relevant serial numbers and software version numbers. Without knowing these, it is impossible to confirm how the device(s) will have behaved. It's also possible that old or obsolete software version numbers will indicate that the systems have not been properly maintained.

   (d) Evidence that the systems are suitable for the clinical purposes for which they are used. If they cannot provide this evidence, then they cannot logically rely on any presumption that the electronic evidence they are using is reliable, Common Law presumptions or otherwise.

   (e) Proportionate evidence of the forensic standards followed, to ensure the integrity of the evidence before and during the investigation. Has the device been used since, or reset? Were there system failures or cyberattacks? Does the data include timestamps? Note, for example, with spreadsheet and simple database data, rows and columns may be edited, duplicated, or deleted without leaving any record of tampering or accidental edits.

   (f) Independent confirmation that the data in fact refers to you or your actions. For instance, in many environments, for historical reasons, there may be multiple staff cards in circulation with your ID on them — so "your" ID may not refer to you.

   (g) The contracts with the digital system suppliers. Contracts often impose unnecessary confidentiality, say that clinical outcomes are a result of your professional judgement, and sometimes even require you to indemnify the manufacturers!

FURTHER READING

🐾 Clinical Human Factors Group (CHFG), https://www.chfg.org
🐾 Health Services Safety Investigations Body (HSSIB), https://www.hssib.org.uk
🐾 National Cyber Security Centre (NCSC), https://www.ncsc.gov.uk
🐾 Institute for Safe Medication Practices (ISMP), https://www.ismp.org

> These four organisations are wonderful resources.

🐾 Marshall, P, Christie, J, Ladkin, PB, Littlewood, B, Mason, S, Newby, M, Rogers, J, Thimbleby, H, & Thomas, M. "Recommendations for the probity of computer evidence," *Digital Evidence and Electronic Signature Law Review*, volume **18**:18–26, 2021. DOI: 10.14296/deeslr.v18i0.5240

> If you're involved in a court case, your lawyers will find this free online article helpful.

🐾 Mason, S & Seng, D (editors). *Electronic Evidence and Electronic Signatures*, OBserving Law, 2021. https://uolpress.co.uk/book/electronic-evidence-and-electronic-signatures DOI: 10.14296/2108.9781911507246

🐾 Ferres, V (Chair), Caddy, CM, Evans, J, Falconer Smith, J & Jones, R. Northern General Hospital NHS Trust, *Report of the Inquiry Committee into the Computer Software Error in Downs Syndrome Screening*, Report submitted on behalf of the inquiry team to the Chief Executive of the Norther General Hospital NHS Trust and The Regional Director of Public Health. Undated.

🐾 Fortson, D & Lintern, S. "NHS spent millions on failed 'AI doctor' app backed by Hancock," *The Sunday Times*, No. 10,389, 29 October, pp 1 & 17–18, 2023.

> This *Sunday Times* article is devastating about Babylon's spectacular failures, and the corruption at the highest levels — a perfect example of Cat Thinking for this booklet! Lots more stuff about Babylon Health can easily be found on the internet.

🐾 NHS. *A just culture guide*, https://www.england.nhs.uk/patient-safety/a-just-culture-guide

🐾 PWC. *Conti cyber attack on the HSE* (redacted), Independent Post Incident Review, Commissioned by the HSE Board in conjunction with the CEO and Executive Management Team, 2021. https://www.hse.ie/eng/services/publications/conti-cyber-attack-on-the-hse-full-report.pdf

🐾 Thimbleby, H & Cairns, P. "Reducing Number Entry Errors: Solving a Widespread, Serious Problem," *Journal Royal Society Interface*, **7**(51):1429–1439, 2010. DOI: 10.1098/rsif.2010.0112

🐾 Thimbleby, H. *Fix IT: See and Solve the Problems of Digital Healthcare*, Oxford University Press, 2021. DOI: 10.1093/oso/9780198861270.001 0001

> Page references to *Fix IT* are provided throughout this booklet. *Fix IT* itself has over 500 notes and references to further material.

🐾 Thimbleby, H. "NHS Number open source software: Implications for digital health regulation and development," *ACM Transactions on Computing for Healthcare*, **3**(4):42:1–42:27, 2022. DOI: 10.1145/3538382

> NHS Numbers are ubiquitous and should be easy to program, so if you're skeptical about how bad healthcare software can be, read this paper. The case study raises the limitations of current digital health standards.

🐾 Wallis, N. *The Great Post Office Scandal*, Bath Publishing, 2021.

ACKNOWLEDGEMENTS

Many thanks to the people whose stories we have shared. Cover photographer Johan B. Skre; illustrator Raden Norfiqri. Some pictures used in this booklet (on the cover, and on pages 2, 4, 5, 9, 17, 19, 20, 21, 22 top, 22 bottom, & 25) were originally published in *Fix IT* on the pages indicated, and have been reproduced by permission of Oxford University Press https://global.oup.com/academic. For permission to reuse material from *Fix IT*, please visit https://global.oup.com/academic/rights

? Why is AI hardly mentioned in this booklet? There are certainly exciting AI stories in the news, but also stories about companies using AI for profit, such as Babylon Health, which as a private company took on patients worldwide but has now gone bust. One affected health authority lost £22 million from Babylon's failure; and two trusts lost £15 million between them when another AI startup, Sensyne Health, collapsed. These huge costs reflect failures of judgement, and affect patient safety, to say nothing of the impact on staff.

The key concern for patient safety is that AI is **far** more complex than other forms of digital, so the engineering problems are far harder. AI developers don't understand exactly how their AI works, AI learns (but who knows exactly what it has learned?), the healthcare systems using it don't understand it, the legal issues (e.g., denying liability) are far more complex, and the companies involved often protect how their systems work for "commercial confidentiality" reasons. And when things go wrong — as they will — AI will be very much harder to understand.

Final thought! We need to prioritise building a new generation of highly skilled digital engineers who can work in or with healthcare to build safe digital healthcare systems.

If you have any questions or suggestions please email us at harold@thimbleby.net

www.ingramcontent.com/pod-product-compliance
Lightning Source LLC
Chambersburg PA
CBHW052046190326
41520CB00003BA/210